Good Cholesterol
Reach A Healthy Blood Pressure Without Drugs

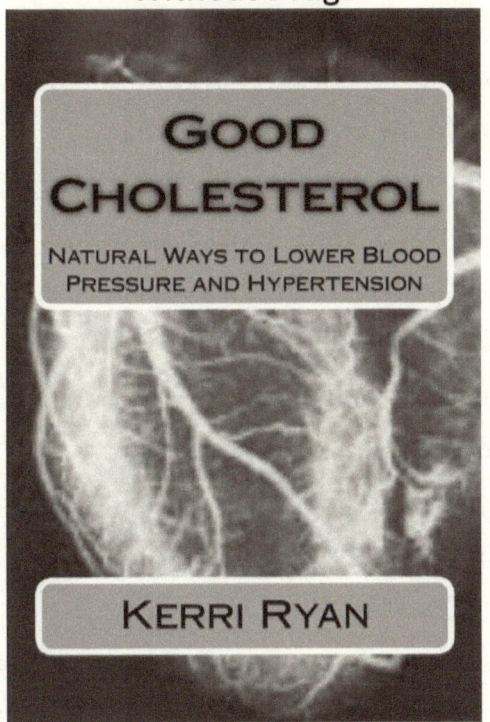

Natural Ways to Improve LDL Cholesterol and Hypertension

By Kerri Ryan
www.Nutritional-Therapy.us

Table of Contents

Cholesterol, Fats, and Oils 3
Signs of Cholesterol Imbalances 7
Basically, Only Three Things 11
Effects of Low Fat Diets 12
The Saturated and Unsaturated Fats 17
Potassium 18
Potassium on a Cellular Level 23
Evolution of Food in America 26
Essential Oils 30
The Results of 35
Adding Lecithin to The Diet 35
Lecithin in Industry 41
Current Trends 42
The Dangers of Low Fat, and Low Cholesterol Diets 43
Metabolic Diseases 45
Summary Diet 46

Cholesterol, Fats, and Oils

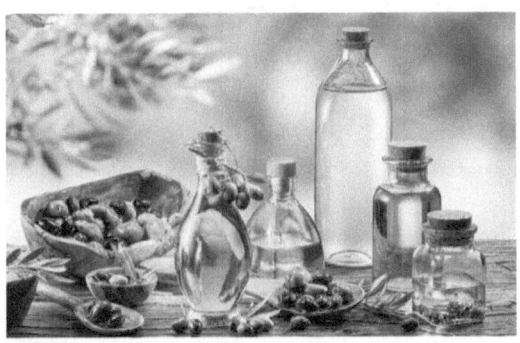

Today, there are few people in America that don't have some kind of cholesterol issues, either too much or too little. It is not responsible to say "Just don't eat so many fats" because the body needs fats and oils to function normally. To remove high fat foods that have so many other nutrients, can be very harmful at best, and dangerous at its worst. Good health is not so much about avoiding foods that have something we don't want; it is about eating other foods that balance each other out. This way the body can process all of it just like it would for anything we eat. It is the lack of nutrition and these nutritional imbalances in the foods we eat that is at the root of so many of the current health issues found in the world today.

Instead of removing food from the diet Nutritional-Therapy.us is advocating that we add other complimentary nutrition so that the body can properly digest and process all foods to their natural end. As Potassium counteracts the effects of salt, Lecithin counteracts the effects of cholesterol, making it perfectly healthy to eat as long as there is a healthy blend of each.

When we have enough lecithin in the diet, the cholesterol in food is broken down completely and will reduce in size to the point that it will be able to get through the arterial walls and make its way to the tissues where it is used by the body. When digested correctly, what is left over breaks down further into carbon dioxide and water, where it is easily excreted from the body.

The body needs a certain amount of cholesterol to function normally, so removing all of it is not feasible, and will only create more problems in the long run[1]. Trying to replace these naturally occurring fats and oils with some sort of man-made substitute will eventually bring a host of side effects that are often worse than having just high blood pressure alone[2].

Everyone needs to find their own healthy cholesterol balance, and give their body what it needs to perform without issues. There is no 'one-size-fits-all' method to a healthy blood pressure, but it can be found as long as the right supplements are taken.

> **'The good news is that the body will be able to find these balances on its own, if the right nutrients are supplied.'**

When the body has enough raw materials, it can process saturated fats like any other substance and excrete the excess without any side effects, or long-term addictions to drugs. It is when cholesterol and essential oils are out of balance that the body naturally looks for ways to get rid of these extra fats that are clogging up the arteries and organs.

As the body is trying to excrete cholesterol it can push it through the skin as with some types of eczema[3], shed them through tears[4], or deposit them somewhere else in the body where they will be out of the way. If the body can't digest and dispose of saturated fats the way it was designed to, this fat will typically store in the arteries causing the infamous cardiovascular disease that is so prevalent in the world today.

By the time you are done with this book you will come to understand what to add to your diet, and why you are adding it. When you understand this, getting back in shape will not be so much of a chore as it is a relief. While many people choose supplements to get their blood pressure under control, it is always best to eat natural and unprocessed food because there are nutrients in them that our bodies need but have not been discovered yet. However, until a person learns how and why to eat naturally, taking supplements will have to do.

Diseases relating to memory disorders such as dementia and Alzheimer's[5]; as well as some muscle disease[6], gallbladder disease[7], liver disease[8], certain types of depression[9], high cholesterol[10], anxiety[11], and certain skin diseases such as eczema[12] are all related to the imbalance of fats and cholesterol. They are all also directly affected by the foods we eat. The goal of this book is to educate the reader about what supplements will make the greatest improvement, and how easily they can accomplish these goals.

Instead of chasing after all the signs and symptoms associated with high cholesterol, the individual can simply reduce all cholesterol build up from the inside out- and reduce or eliminate these issues by addressing the real problem; undigested saturated fats. Why would anyone take handfuls of expensive prescription drugs that will make them more drug dependent, when they can add certain nutrients to the diet and cause them to melt these fats away from the inside out?

Why would someone take drugs that offer only a limited amount of time for improvement until the side effects start to manifest? Or make them more drug dependent?
Because most people simply don't know any other way.
This demographic also includes many well-meaning doctors, too. While diet and nutrition affect most diseases that the human body can experience, this publication will be focusing only on high cholesterol and blood pressure, and the supplements that will correct it. However, don't be surprised if a few other health issues disappear along the way.

Signs of Cholesterol Imbalances

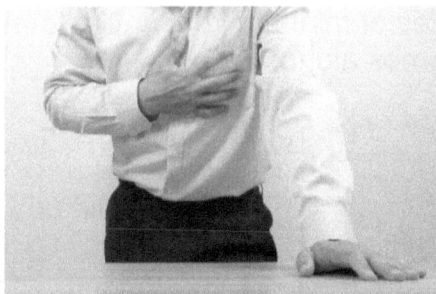

Blockage in the Heart- As you are probably already aware, saturated fat is readily stored in and along arterial walls throughout the body, gradually narrowing the blood vessels until they become completely blocked. Once blood flow is

completely cut off, those blood vessels will seize, and the cells around them will begin to die from a lack of oxygen. If not reversed immediately, these occurrences can be permanent, or even fatal.
When this constriction takes place in the heart, it starts out as angina, and if left unchecked will develop into a full-fledged heart attack.

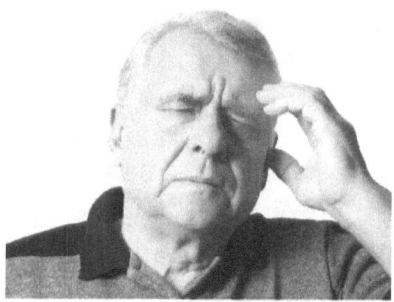

Blockage in the Brain- When salt is retained, and/or saturated fats begin to build up in the blood vessels of the brain, these people start to have an occasional series of headaches and random sharp pains here and there, eventually progressing to more frequent bouts of confusion. If left unchecked this will progress to a series of mini-strokes, until a fatal one eventually comes along.

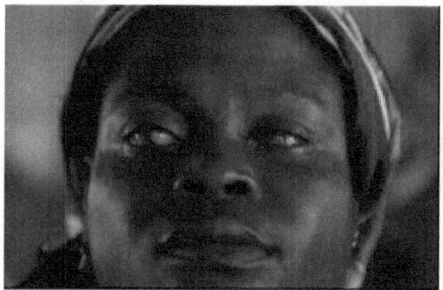

Blockage in the Eyes- Fatty build up in and around the vessels in the eyes can lead to cataracts[13]

and small, yellow fatty deposits shed through tearing and watery eyes. This is an attempt to rid the body of excess fat. Reducing the size of the fat molecules in the blood is the best way to effectively slow down and begin reversing cataracts from forming and progressing.

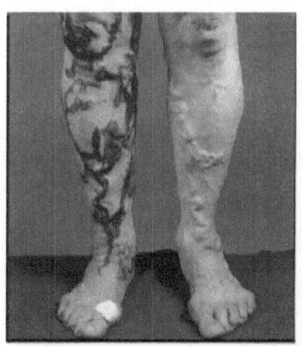

Blockage in the Legs- Saturated fat built up in the legs can limit blood flow, causing poor circulation, varicose veins, and pain that can be so severe that it used to lead to amputation some years ago.

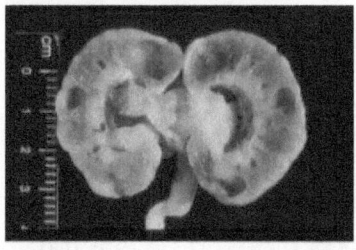

Blockages in the Kidneys- If fatty deposits build up in the in the kidneys it can lead to nephritis. Once this takes place, this person will surely be under the direct and closely monitored care of a specialist as kidney failure is usually one of the last steps before death.

No matter how you look at it, a buildup of saturated fats and cholesterol anywhere in the body will always have a negative effect on the person in general, and ridding the body of it is a must in order to live a normal, healthy life. Despite what some experts say, heart disease is not permanent; it is reversible without using drugs, once you learn to see the overall picture. Prescription drugs such as clot-busters play a vital role in taking control over an emergency situation, but they are in no means a permanent solution to a long-term problem.

So, when your doctor tells you that high blood pressure cannot be cured, only managed with the use of statins and other drugs realize that this is only his understanding, and not endorsed by those outside of his medical community. Nutritional-Therapy has seen hundreds of people successfully reverse and eliminate high blood pressure apart from drug use, and they do this without any side effects at all. All these various conditions; coronary disease, stroke, cataracts, varicose veins, cataracts and nephritis all stem from the same fundamental problem. If cholesterol is not being broken down during digestion it is left to roam around in the body and deposit wherever it can.

Once these fats are broken down into smaller particles, people will begin to see how easy it is to reduce cholesterol buildup and return blood cholesterol levels back to normal just by adding a few things to your existing diet. These build ups didn't happen overnight, so they will not return overnight either. However, if the person stays with it, and continues to supplement their diet with the right nutrients, they will begin to notice their body taking strides towards a stronger, healthier position in a matter of a few months.

It is not uncommon for people to feel the expulsion of these lingering saturated fat build-ups melt away from inside them, as they are being moved out of the body. Eventually, over time the individual that stays with their regimen of supplements will regain the health they once knew in younger years and find that their doctor will tell them that they don't need to continue taking their BP meds anymore since their blood results show a vast improvement.

Basically, Only Three Things

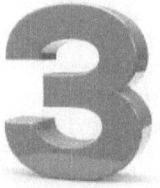

There are basically only three things that will affect someone's blood pressure.

1. Cholesterol that narrows arteries and veins restricting blood flow
2. Salt that will retain water
3. Lack of Choline that facilitates chemical reactions

In this reading, this is what we will focus on and this is what you can expect to change your blood pressure back to normal. There are other factors of course, such as losing weight, but losing weight alone will not lower your blood pressure. Lowering blood pressure is a chemical process that will take place once the body has what it needs to balance the bodies chemistry.

Effects of Low Fat Diets

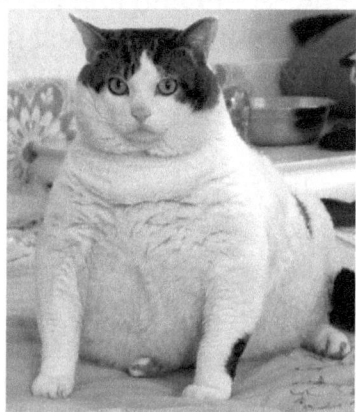

Simply removing all fats is reckless and dangerous, and should not be a part of any long term treatment[14]. Fats take longer to digest, so they make us feel full longer. Without them people tend to eat far more calories from sugars and starches instead. Ironically, these calories[15] are quickly converted into body fat, and will cause the blood fat and cholesterol levels to spike once again.[16] Low fat diets typically end up with three negative results;

1. These fat and cholesterol particles from calories and sugars increase significantly in size[17], making them that much more difficult to exit the arterial walls.
2. It has also been found that the amount of blood cholesterol from starches that is converted into bile acids is also significantly decreased[18], making the individuals overall condition much worse[19] than if they had just eaten some foods that contain a small amount of fat.
3. These low-fat diets will also throw the liver into overdrive and cause it to produce far more cholesterol than it would under different conditions. This causes the blood cholesterol level to rise sharply yet again.[20]

Low fat diets more often than not produce exactly the opposite of what heart disease patients want to achieve, yet some doctors are still prescribing them to their patients since they just don't know any different.

The body needs cholesterol, so it is not realistic to remove it all. The key is to ingest it with other counterbalancing elements will make it easy for the body to process them just like anything else we eat.

Some forms of cholesterol are used for proper adrenal and sex hormone function, proper pituitary gland function, and some cholesterol is even converted to vitamin D when the skin is exposed to sunlight.[21] When combined with bile acids, cholesterol also helps to digest and absorb food all through the small intestine so that we can actually benefit from what we eat. So, you can see all cholesterols were not created equal, and they are not all inherently bad.

Fats are graded or categorized based on their hydrogen content.[22] Saturated fats are known by chemistry buffs as single bonded carbon chains. Unsaturated fats are double and triple bonded carbon chains;[23] as seen in the next image;

Saturated Fatty Acid

Unsaturated Fatty Acid

For the layman, saturated fats are fats that are solid at room temperature such as animal fats and butter; unsaturated fats are fats that are liquid at room temperature such as fish oil, soy and vegetable oils.

In order to lower saturated fats in the blood, Lecithin needs to be added and foods with unsaturated fats should be eaten. Unsaturated fats are the double and triple bonded carbon chains in the picture above. The double and triple bonds of the unsaturated fats will break up the single bonds of the saturated fats and dilute them so to speak, reducing them in size so that they can be moved out of the arteries and on to the tissues and organs for practical use.

Patients with low blood pressure are always found to have small particles of unsaturated fats in their blood, while persons with high blood pressure are always found with large particles of saturated fat in their blood.[24] The result is that these large particles begin to build up, form plaque, and eventually shut off that artery. The good news is that the individual can start to reverse this situation starting today simply by adding unsaturated fats back into their diet and/or taking Lecithin.

It is not so much about removing fats as it is about adding unsaturated fats so that the body can process everything through the digestive system. Apart from an emergency situation, if we try to remove fats some other way, there is a high risk of creating another problem somewhere else.

So, follow your doctor's orders if you are under one's care, but if not, then the next time you are eating a big juicy hamburger just take some Lecithin and/or wheat germ with it. This will break up the fats and allow them to keep moving through the body fluidly without causing any undue stress to the cardiovascular system.

The Saturated and Unsaturated Fats

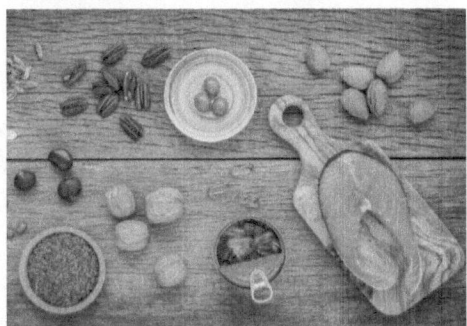

There is so much talk about fats, oils, saturated and unsaturated...It is difficult to keep up with it all. The key thing to understand is the saturated fats are bad, because they are saturated with hydrogen, and clog up the arteries, while unsaturated fats are good because they break the bonds of saturated fats, and make them easier for the body to digest. It is the same thing with high density lipids, and low-density lipids,[25] where Low Density or LDL's, and the saturated fats, and HDL's are unsaturated. You say Tomato, I say Tomah-to. The bottom line is these single bonded carbon chains need to have their bonds broken so the body can wash them away. The best way to do this, is start eating more of a plant-based diet, as these foods will have far more nutrients than any supplement will have.

Unprocessed food has elements in them that we have not even identified yet. However, if you are like me, and can't stand the taste of rutabagas and parsnips no matter how they are prepared, then there is an alternative. Lecithin and Wheat germ will start to break down these fats immediately, and over the first few weeks, many people can actually feel them washing though your body on their way out.

Potassium

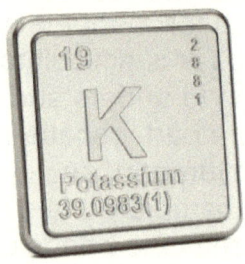

The next key element in lowering blood pressure is Potassium. While Lecithin will lower cholesterol and help to open up the vessels, Potassium with help to lower the Blood Pressure by allowing the kidneys and the chemistry of the blood to regulate itself by flushing away salts that retain water.

I want to preface this chapter by saying that if your doctor has you on Digitalis, speak with him first before you start adding Potassium to your diet.

High blood pressure can be created in volunteers simply by adding so much salt, that the body uses up all its potassium trying to get rid of it, thus creating a potassium deficiency. It is not enough to just lower salt intake, Potassium needs to be added to complete the chemical reaction.

Whether too much salt, or not enough potassium, so much water can be retained in the blood that the pressure can rise significantly in minutes. There is a lot of study on cholesterol as related to high blood pressure, but not so much study about potassium and high blood pressure, and yet it plays a major role in regulating it. Around the world, cultures with high blood pressure invariably have a high salt diet; but it is unheard of in societies with low salt diets, or diets high in potassium.

Take Japan as an example. Before these things were better understood heart disease in Japan was rare, but brain hemorrhaging brought on my high blood pressure was the leading cause of death back in the 1970's.[26] Northern Japan eats primarily salted fish, with an average of 27 grams of salt daily, leading to a much higher instance of brain hemorrhaging than takes place in the South, where they eat approximately 17 grams daily. Similarly, in

America, those with high blood pressure average a 4-20 grams salt intake daily; and the tissues of American stroke victims have a much higher salt content than those who die of other causes. Lower salt intake has been used for decades as a means to lower blood pressure, but because severe salt restrictions can be dangerous, this approach may not be the best one alone. Adding Potassium to the diet is a far better way to lower water retention that contributes to high blood pressure.

The kidneys are the organ that actually regulate blood pressure, so getting them healthy is a good place to start. After starting the practice of cleaning out the saturated fat with Lecithin and Wheat Germ, regulating their salt and potassium balance is the next step. Lowering the blood volume is another way to lower the blood pressure once the vessels start to open up.

The kidneys are lined with thousands of tiny tubules in order to provide lots of surface area where chemical reactions can take place. This is far better designed to detect these salt/potassium balances much better than we can by just checking the blood pressure externally. This is why healthy kidneys have a great deal to do with a healthy blood pressure.

Since salt retains water, we need to find a safe way to balance the salt intake with potassium, so the kidneys can regulate the blood pressure and keep it under control. It is not enough to simply remove salt; the body needs potassium to complete the chemical reactions. Again, it is not so much about what we need to remove from our diets, but what we need to add to our diets in order to balance out the blood chemistry. Removing sodium altogether can bring other issues that we won't go into here, so simply said, by adding Potassium, this will cause the body to lose salt and water through the kidneys safely without any sudden drops, thereby lowering the overall blood pressure without issue.

There are a few other elements that will help to rid the body of salt and lower the blood pressure apart from simply removing it from the diet.

1. Calcium and Vitamin D also help to spill salt in the urine[27]
2. Since readers are already taking Lecithin to rid the body of cholesterol, this cholesterol will be pushed up to the surface of the skin. When this happens, sitting in the sun for as little as 1-hour per day will convert this cholesterol into a safe and natural form of Vitamin D.

This is probably the best option for most people.[28]
3. Lab rats with high blood pressure caused by a salt toxicity have been known to recover once they are given healthy amounts of the water-soluble B-vitamins, in particular Choline and Pantothenic Acid[29]

Sodium and potassium are constantly balancing back and forth in the blood, causing one or the other to be lost into the urine. People who ate as much salt as they liked excreted 9 times more potassium in the urine than those who restricted salt use.[30] Other volunteers who were denied potassium retained so much salt that they developed high blood pressure without having signs of it before.[31] This is also the reason why animals that eat a high Potassium diet of leaves and grass, will walk hundreds of miles just to get some salt from a salt-block placed in some random field. Nature is always seeking to balance salt and potassium within the blood. The body knows what it needs and what it must do, all we must do is give it the raw materials and the body will self-correct on its own.

When potassium is ingested, whether through food or a supplement, high blood pressure will return to normal provided that the only cause of high blood pressure was too much salt. If the cause of high blood pressure was plaque built up, the Lecithin will work on that. Between the two, Lecithin and Potassium, the body will be able to open the arteries and balance the pressure by itself, without side effects, and without a chemical dependency that so many suffer from while on a diet of prescription drugs.

Potassium on a Cellular Level

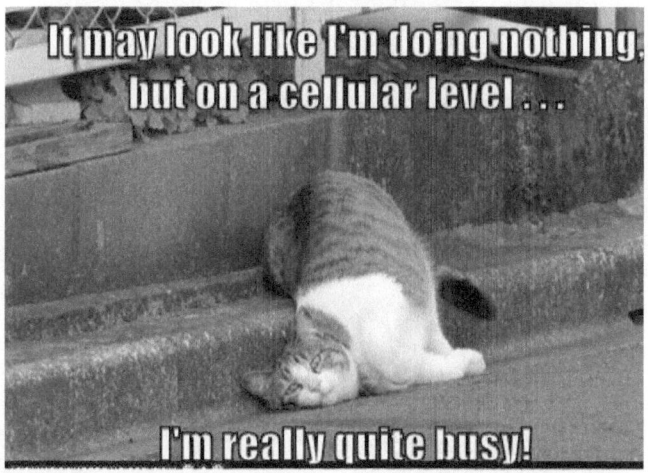

Under normal conditions, potassium remains inside the cells, while salt remains in the fluid around them. Because of this, both sodium and potassium play a key role in regulating the contents of not just the overall blood pressure, but of each individual cell pressure as well. When the potassium level inside the cells decreases, sodium enters in and brings so much fluid that the cell becomes water logged.[32] This is the reason why so many high blood pressure patients also experience Oedema, also known as Dropsy.[33]

Typically, between 5-15 grams of potassium chloride throughout the day will do as much if not more to reduce blood pressure than just restricting salt. Mostly because we are not even aware of how much salt we are eating since it is in almost everything we eat. Trying to reduce intake is far more challenging than simply adding the suggested potassium chloride. You will know if you are taking too much is you start to experience;

1. nausea
2. vomiting
3. upset stomach
4. gas
5. diarrhea
6. tingling in your hands or feet[34]

Don't take any potassium is you are taking Digitalis- Speak with your doctor first as this will be a delicate balance.

It is always best to add supplements slowly a take notice of how your body reacts to them no matter what they are. Even though supplements are "natural", if taking them by the handful without knowing what they will do, this can be dangerous and make you feel sick. Like the B-Vitamins, never take them on an empty stomach. They won't hurt you, but they will make you extremely nauseous.

There are too many influencing factors between each individual to make a blanket statement about taking supplements, but simply note that Potassium Chloride supplements will actively lower blood pressure far more than just restricting salt,[35] and at the same time you need to be aware of when enough is enough.

Diets consisting of rice, fruit and sugar are often prescribed to help reduce salt, but these foods are almost completely void of any nutrition. They have almost no B vitamins, Vitamin E or complete proteins. However, if you can endure this diet for a few months, it has been known to reduce blood pressure.

When foods are overcooked or refined, they lose most of their original value. Plus, Americans rarely eat fresh fruits and vegetables anymore, so it is easy to see why blood pressure issues are so epidemic. These nutritionally void practices combined with the excessive urinary losses of potassium have now caused a fairly wide spread potassium deficiency in our culture. Both sodium and potassium should be in the diet, and in the correct balance in order to maintain a good blood pressure. Assuming the kidneys are healthy, they will know what to do with the foods we eat, and when given the correct raw materials, our bodies will self-correct in a very short time.

Evolution of Food in America

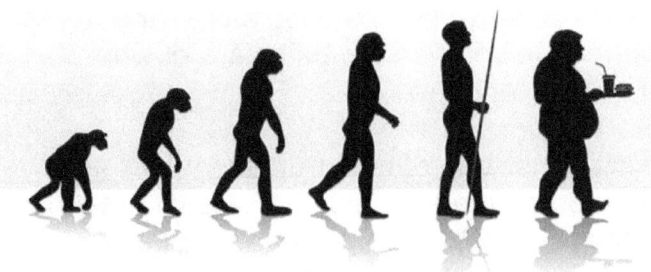

One of the biggest changes that we have seen in this generation over the last 70 years is the mass production of food. Most of us are already well versed on the evils of fast food, but food bought in the grocery stores can be just as bad. 'Super-markets' are a relatively new phenomenon.[36] Before the 1950's there were very few large 'super' markets that distributed so much food, or even the variety of food that we see today. Once the larger suburban markets started to spring up across the country, the demand for volume and variety skyrocketed. In order to meet these demands, the mass produced, genetically modified, processed food niche began to take shape.

Foods started to be cut with fillers and preservatives, and any part of a food that would cause it to spoil was quickly stripped away in exchange for a longer shelf life.[37] Ironically, the portion of the food that causes it to spoil is the very portion that the human body needs the most in order to stay healthy. Bread for example, was historically made from the whole grain, including the husk. Today, the wheat germ, that portion that contains 22 nutritional elements and is basically the 'storehouse of the grain', is stripped out and sold separately. Even if the bread says 'whole grain', if it doesn't need to be refrigerated, it won't contain any wheat germ because that would spoil in just a few days. Because of the nuances in the law, manufactures can legally call their products 'whole grain bread', even when the wheat germ has been taken out.

See Dr. Oz's personal endorsement of this Super Food we call Wheat Germ, to see just how much nutrition we are missing.

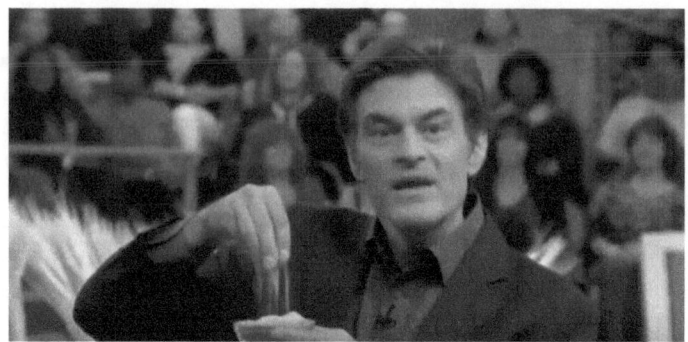

https://youtu.be/i3UiG0VpVl4

Ironically, white bread without the germ started to really be mass-produced back in the 1940's when soldiers were returning from World War II.[38] There was a huge need to mass-produce everything, and Wonder bread lead the way with their bleached white bread pumped full of air. Once that started, the United States started seeing a huge increase in Pellagra and heart disease.[39] As time went by, research showed that white bread contained almost no nutrition and was starting to deprive American's of their main source of all the B-vitamins, essential oils and Lecithin.

Without the B-vitamins, specifically Niacin, people will develop Pellagra,[40] and without the emulsifier Lecithin, saturated fats are not broken down properly so they get 'stuck' in the arteries and veins causing cardiovascular disease. Lecithin is the body's greatest defense against high blood pressure and heart disease. Without wheat germ people are losing one of the largest sources of these 2 nutrients, and many others in their diet.

Once this became well known the FDA started to require that in order for a food to be called 'bread', it must contain 'Eight Essential Vitamins and Minerals'.[41] So, what did bread manufactures do? They stripped out all of the nutrition; put back a small portion of it and rebranded their product as 'Enriched'.

The 'nutritional value' aspect of food became incidental when compared to profits, and sadly the American people have since been fed 'food-stuffs' with little nutritional value at all, along with a huge portion of misinformation on the side. We are seeing today far more nutritionally based diseases in all age groups, which were rarely heard of before the 1950's.

Cataracts,[42] Juvenile diabetes,[43] arthritis,[44] atherosclerosis,[45] and even cancer[46] are relatively common in children today, and yet practically unheard of 70 years ago; all of which can be directly related to diet and nutrition. To be competitive in the food industry, one of the main elements manufacturers must have is a long shelf life. You must be able to have your product available on the shelves for a reasonable amount of time, or the market won't carry it. One-way to extend the life of food is to remove those naturally occurring parts of it that cause it to spoil. Oils in particular will turn rancid relatively quickly, so many of these have been replaced with 'hydrogenated' oils, causing unsaturated fats to become saturated so they would last longer.[47] Once this chemical reaction has taken place, these foods that brought nourishment and health to our bodies turned into foods that caused hardening of the arteries and all the associated diseases that tag along with it.[48]

Essential Oils

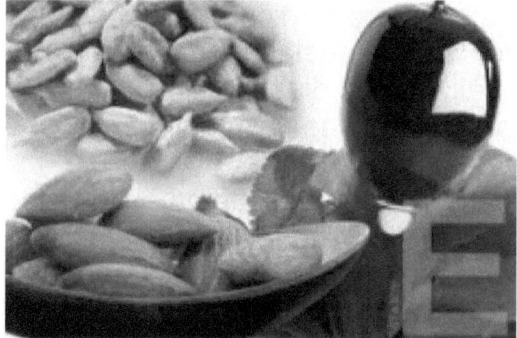

The liver will produce its own Lecithin and help to keep these fats and oils in check, but it needs a few raw materials to get the job done. Any nutrients that will help produce Lecithin will ultimately help to alleviate and reverse heart disease as well as all the other cholesterol-based diseases; however, the three main essential oils in the diet are;

1. Arachidonic Acid[49]
2. Linoleic Acid[50]
3. Linolenic Acid[51]

This is probably more information than most people need to know so don't get too caught up in it, however, not surprisingly, saturated fats like animal fats and butter contain little or no essential fatty acids.[52] The fatty acid **Arachidonic** is necessary before Lecithin can be utilized properly, and the more Arachidonic acid there is in the blood of animals, the more resistant they are to atherosclerosis.[53] Additionally, when these same animals are given the three essential oils together, they all showed an increase in blood Lecithin almost immediately.[54]

When the vegetable oil **Linoleic** is given to test animals, the cholesterol in the blood is changed into bile salts much quicker;[55] and the conversion of cholesterol into carbon dioxide and water within the tissues takes place much faster as well.[56] *Linoleic acid*, or omega-6 fatty acid, and *linolenic acid*, or omega-3 fatty acid, are the two essential fatty acids. They are considered as essential because the body cannot synthesize them and needs to obtain them from the diet. A lack of either one will prevent the body from maintaining good health, and sooner or later, symptoms will start to develop.[57]

It takes so little oil to meet the bodies' requirements, only about one to two tablespoons a day will keep normal blood cholesterol stable, but simply swallowing this amount directly without the other required nutrition will have little effect on the overall cholesterol levels.[58] Lecithin is still needed to attack cholesterol problems effectively.
These oils are only part of the chemical makeup of Lecithin, and that is why they are important to include in the daily diet, but these oils alone will not reduce cholesterol.
This is a good example of why it is best to eat natural, unprocessed foods. There are things in whole foods that we have not isolated yet, so by eating the whole food in its natural state, we are sure to get everything Nature intended to ensure good health and stable blood cholesterol and pressure.

There is nothing inherently wrong with saturated fat as long as the cells are supplied with enough of all the other nutrients needed to utilize them. The need for these nutrients is of course proportional to the amount of fats being eaten. So, the next time someone tries to explain these oils as if they are the answer to all cholesterol problems just remember that they are only part of a bigger picture. Remember that these oils alone do little to address any existing saturated fat already on arterial walls. Therefore, it is recommended that cholesterol issues be addressed first with Lecithin, and this way the essential oils will then compliment this primary dietary change.

The fish oils that are so popular today ironically have no essential fatty acids, but will help to reduce cholesterol by decreasing the body's ability to absorb it.[59] Like the essential oils, they will also not do anything to address existing plaque buildup. It is also important to remember that oils contain about 100 calories per tablespoon and any of these calories not burned for fuel will typically store in the body as flabby fat, such as seen behind the arms and below the chin.

Avoiding saturated fat is usually a good thing, especially since we American's tend to eat way too much of it. However, remember that adding Lecithin will do far more than just reducing fats. Ultimately, it is better to start by adding Lecithin to the diet, rather than trying to eliminate more fats from the diet. Eliminating fats from the diet will consequently limit several other healthy nutrients that are needed now more than ever to restore a balanced blood cholesterol, and more importantly, good health.

In summary, during digestion, fats in general are broken down into what are collectively known as fatty acids.[60] These acids include both saturated and unsaturated fatty acids, together comprising the fats. They are graded based on their hydrogen content.[61] It is when these are out of balance that atherosclerosis begins to form. When people talk about fats, the current talk is about good HDL's and bad HDL's, but basically this is trying to make the distinction between saturated and unsaturated fats, and then to what degree.

Finding the balance between these two fatty acids is the way to bring atherosclerosis under control, no matter how severe it is. Not to be redundant, but this is most effectively done by adding Lecithin to the diet. It can be purchased at any nutrition center such as GNC and/or taken in the form of Wheat Germ. Wheat germ has so many other excellent nutrients in it, no matter what heath issue you are dealing with, Wheat Germ should be a part of everyone's daily diet.[62] Better yet, take both. They are natural and won't contraindicate any pharmaceuticals someone might be taking. You can't take too much, but always check with your physician before making any changes since every individual is unique.

The Results of Adding Lecithin to The Diet

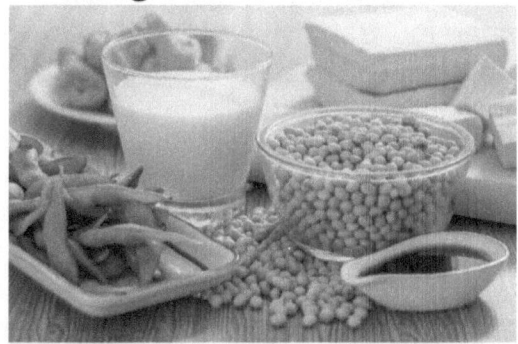

Like cholesterol, Lecithin is continuously being produced by a healthy liver. With the help of bile acids, Lecithin is then absorbed by the blood.[63] Because Lecithin is an emulsifier, it will aid in the movement of fats throughout the entire body, in particular those small arteries and veins as are found in the eyes and lungs. Most importantly, Lecithin will support the removal of fats and cholesterols out of the blood, and on to the tissues where it can be used properly.[64]

Another important thing Lecithin does is assist The bile acids in utilizing existing cholesterol in the body during digestion, thereby further reducing the amounts of cholesterol found in the blood.[65]

Lecithin will also play a role in the structural make up of every cell in the body, particularly the brain and nervous system.[66] In a healthy person, Lecithin makes up as much as 30% of the dry weight on the brain, and 73% of the total liver fat; both of which are greatly diminished in those dying of heart disease.[67]

Lecithin is a powerful emulsifying agent in both medicine and industry, and vital to preventing and correcting cardio-vascular disease no matter what stage the disease has progressed to. While low fat diets and adding unsaturated fats back into the diet is generally considered 'a good thing', they won't address existing heart disease alone. It takes Lecithin to see more noticeable and lasting results.[68]

Blood is fundamentally a water solution into which fats cannot dissolve. If Lecithin is present and in healthy amounts, and with the help of bile acids, Lecithin will cause cholesterol and other fats to be broken down into much smaller particles so they can be held in suspension. This way they will be able to pass out of the blood, and on to the tissues for good use.[69]

Studies have revealed that all atherosclerosis patients are characterized by an increase in blood cholesterol, and a decrease in Lecithin.[70] It was shown as early as 1935, that experimental heart disease can be produced and controlled by increasing cholesterol, and reducing Lecithin in the diet.[71] In addition to this, with enough Lecithin present, heart disease will not occur no matter how much cholesterol is fed.[72] Even in cases of advanced heart disease, conditions improved dramatically after Lecithin is added.[73] Some of these findings have also shown that;

1. Lab animals that have the ability to produce their own Lecithin have a much greater ability to resist heart disease than animals that do not have this capability.[74]
2. In the liver of a healthy person, Lecithin will immediately start to produce in generous amounts once a fatty meal has been eaten. It will then travel directly to the bloodstream where it will begin to change these larger fat particles into much smaller ones once the fat and Lecithin is combined there.[75]
3. In cardio-vascular diseased individuals their blood Lecithin will remain low regardless of the amount of fat entering the blood. The end result is that the saturated fat particles remain too large to pass through the arterial walls, so they sit there in the arteries and begin to accumulate.[76]

This lack of Lecithin will not only allow heart

disease to continue, but the lack of Lecithin in the individual's cells and their structural integrity is even more damaging to the central nervous system. There needs to be more study on this, but Lecithin is known to rebuild the Myelin Sheath surrounding each and every nerve cell, particularly in the brain and spinal cord. It is believed that by rebuilding this Myelin Sheath with Lecithin, many Alzheimer's and Multiple Sclerosis patients, and those who suffer from the effects of a stroke will be able to regain more mobility and muscle function and at faster rates.[77]

Still more studies have shown that when the bile duct of experimental animals was tied, to prevent any further cholesterol from the liver to enter the blood, and a solution of Lecithin was allowed to flow continuously into the arteries of these test animals, even severe atherosclerosis with hardened plaque deposits was quickly and efficiently washed away.[78]

In addition to this, if the body's cholesterol supply is cut off and injections of Lecithin are given, the blood cholesterol increases, proving that existing cholesterol is being broken down and washed away from where ever it is being stored elsewhere in the body.[79]

There is more than enough evidence to prove that Lecithin is the key to reducing cholesterol and plaque, however, there is so much money to be made with pharmaceuticals that this information is prevented from being widely known. It is unfortunately becoming all too common that those who make this nutritional information available will often and suddenly and for reasons unknown, have a very unfortunate accident… Truth can be dangerous.

These are just a few reasons why a complete and balanced diet that includes nutritional supplements are so important. Cholesterol can be produced from fat, sugar, and even indirectly from proteins. So, trying to starve yourself in the hope of not eating anything with fats or oils in it will actually have the reverse effect you are trying to achieve. As stated before, lowering cholesterol is not so much about taking foods out of our diets, as it is adding those nutrients that will help to reduce and process cholesterol out of our bodies.

When I refer to the 'right supplements', I am referring to ones manufactured in a quality lab; and not a cheap, low dose, 'make you feel better' brand sold within dollar stores. This is certainly better than nothing, but if you are serious about improving your health to the point that you will be able to wean yourself off prescription drugs, then you will need to make a concentrated effort along with some investment. In the nutritional supplement industry, there are far more 'profit making' supplements than there are 'result producing' ones. You Get What You Pay For.

By adding the essential fatty acids and the B vitamins choline and inositol to the diet, this will directly help to build the structural make up of Lecithin within the body and thereby support the whole 'anti-atherosclerosis' scenario. Lecithin is essential for the form and function of literally every cell in the body. A lack of any one of these nutritional elements can compromise the body's health in several ways, and contribute to the advancement of many diseases besides cardiovascular. If patients do nothing else but purchase a Lecithin supplement and start taking 3-4 capsules at every meal, this is a good start to reversing atherosclerosis, supporting proper brain and nervous system function, and a giant step forward in the right direction.

Lecithin in Industry

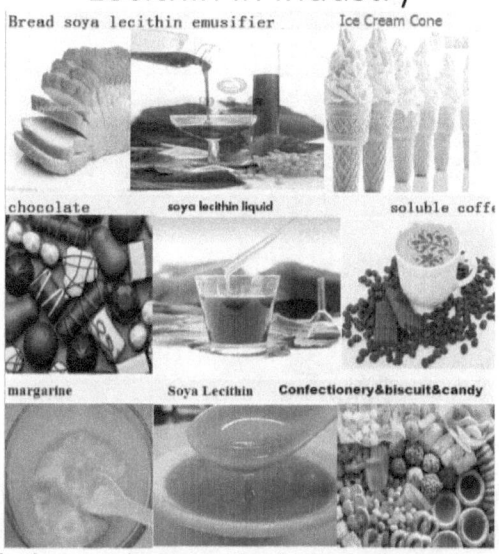

Lecithin is used extensively in industry, too. Because it can be oily, it is removed from vegetable oil in the making of paint. This lecithin by-product is sold in granular form yet is still a viable and potent source. In the baking industry, Lecithin will convert fats into small particles, acting as an emulsifying agent producing a smoother tasting end product. This is one reason why we are starting to hear stories about how chocolate is good for the heart. However, I doubt that the little bit of Lecithin used to make a candy bar hardly justifies eating all the other sugars and fats that go along with it. Nonetheless, whether this Lecithin comes from eggs, liver, nuts, wheat germ, soy, or chocolate; heart disease patients will benefit from Lecithin, no matter its source.[80]

Current Trends

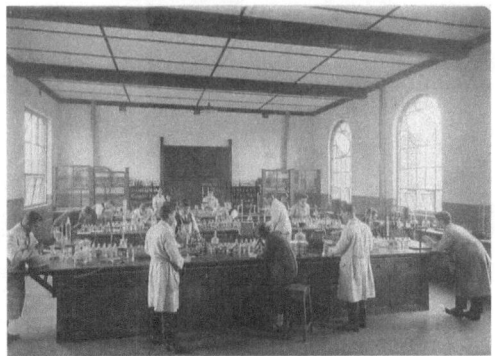

Many physicians are just now starting to rediscover the restorative benefits of Lecithin even though results have been around since the 1930's.[81] Because of the tremendous profitability of pharmaceutical drugs, statins in particular, this information is being aggressively denied for several reasons.
The facts remain; when 4-6 tablespoons of Lecithin were given daily to atherosclerosis patients; including heart and cerebral atherosclerosis, all experienced improvement; without exception.

Even those with advanced heart disease lasting as long as ten years, and found to be resistant to drug therapy, even these patients found themselves improving day by day.[82] Within one to three months without any other dietary changes, all these patients' blood cholesterol levels dropped sharply when given Lecithin. Patients felt more energetic, were able to go back to work again, and were relieved of any pain, signs or symptoms.[83] After their recoveries, one to two tablespoons of Lecithin daily helped to maintain healthy blood cholesterol levels indefinitely.[84]

The Dangers of Low Fat, and Low Cholesterol Diets

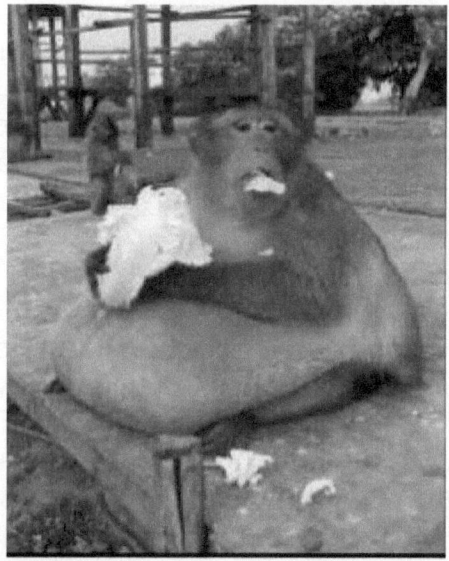

These diets are largely considered dangerous by those in alternative medicine as they have been from the 1960's.[85] Many of these 'restricted' foods are full of the exact nutrients needed to utilize the fats associated with heart disease.

Mayonnaise is a good example. It averages 52-67% essential fatty acids, and 10 to 14% Lecithin.[86] Eggs are another excellent food source that have been attacked as unhealthy despite their high Lecithin and high methionine levels.[87] Volunteers recovering from heart attacks have been found that after eating 10 eggs, 16 egg yolks, and even as much as 60 grams of pure cholesterol daily for varying periods of time, their cholesterol did not rise at all as long as the eggs were not cooked in saturated fat.[88] Despite the high cholesterol content, eggs contain even higher levels of Lecithin, negating the effects of the cholesterol. They also contain so many other nutritional Elements that taking them out of the diet does far more harm than good.

Butter is another villain that doesn't get the credit it deserves. When it is eaten with a generally poor diet, it will absolutely raise cholesterol levels across the board. However, persons in Denmark, Switzerland and Finland eat far more butterfat than we do here in the States, and yet have much less heart disease than we do in America.[89] How can this be?

People in parts of Africa eat as much as 60 to 65% of their calories from butter fat, but because the rest of their diet is unrefined and full of natural fruits and vegetables, heart disease is virtually unheard of as they enjoy an average of 125 milligrams of blood cholesterol per person.[90]

Even here in America, our grandparents and great-grandparents would slather butter on everything they could eat; yet heart disease was not nearly as prevalent prior to World War II as it is today. The natural conclusion would be that it is not cholesterol alone that is the problem here, but rather the lack of the other nutrients needed to effectively utilize it, and then process any extra out of the body.

Metabolic Diseases

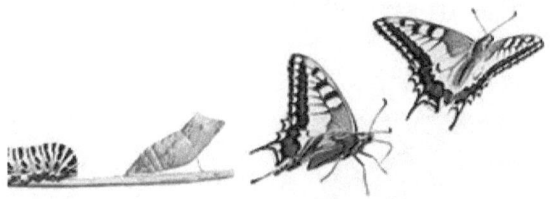

Heart disease is a metabolic disease, defined As *'...affected by metabolism'*, and *'undergoing metamorphosis'*[91]

So metabolic diseases are by their very definition always changing, and never permanent. So, you can see that since heart disease is a metabolic disease, it is clearly not permanent. Just as it can evolve into a more dangerous state, it can also evolve into a less dangerous state, depending on the foods we eat. Metabolic diseases are those that change slowly over time, as compared to infectious or contagious diseases that are transmitted readily through the air or by physical contact. The fact is that all metabolic diseases are directly affected by diet and nutrition; including, high cholesterol, diabetes, arthritis, and even many forms of cancer. So, when your doctor tells you that your high cholesterol and high blood pressure is permanent, and that all you can do is manage it, he is misinformed. Take into consideration that he probably got his medical degree 20-40 years ago and got it from a school that was funded by a pharmaceutical company. Step outside of the box and learn something new.

Summary Diet

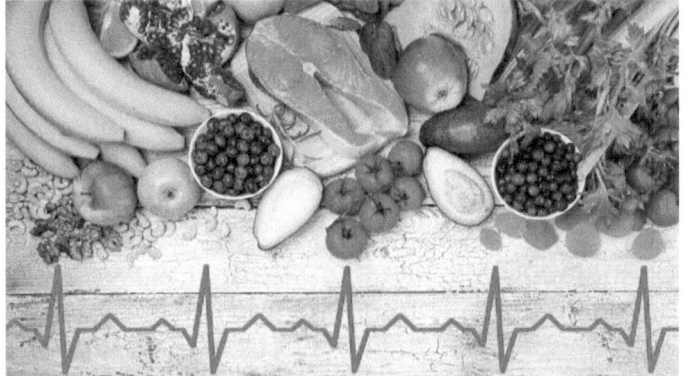

In summary, the goal here is not just to lower blood pressure and cholesterol in order to win the coveted 120/80, but to repair the heart, kidneys, brain and vision; to bring everything back into balance recreating the smooth running machine that the body was meant to be. What good will mountains of drugs and caffeine do if the overall body is slowly sliding downhill? Treat your body right, and it will serve you well throughout your life. The suggested servings for a good cholesterol /sodium/ potassium balance should be as follows;

1. A source of essential fatty acids, and the B vitamins choline and inositol.
2. A minimum of 3-6 (21) grain capsules of Lecithin daily, or 2-3 with each meal
3. 2-4 tablespoons of Wheat Germ daily, or 1-2 tablespoons with each meal.
4. A B-complex vitamin that includes all the B's, and/or 1-2 bottles of Vitamin Water each day.
5. A fresh source of protein such as bananas, other fruits and vegetables as often as you can, and/or a protein shake. 35 grams of protein a day is the average.
6. A salt substitute, consisting of Potassium chloride and salt, or adding 250 mg of Potassium to each meal. However, speak with your doctor before adding Potassium if you are taking Digitalis-

Also, leave a review on our web site,
www.Nutritional-Therapy.us

Thank you for sharing us on Facebook!
https://www.facebook.com/NutritionalTherapyUS/

www.Nutritional-Therapy.us
NutritionalTherapyUS@gmail.com

[1] http://www.health.harvard.edu/topics/cholesterol ; http://www.hopkinsmedicine.org/news/media/releases/statin_use_linked_to_rare_autoimmune_muscle_disease_study_finds
[2] http://www.hopkinsmedicine.org/news/media/releases/statin_use_linked_to_rare_autoimmune_muscle_disease_study_finds
[3] Gross, P., et al, NY State Journal of Med 50, 2683, 1950
[4] Vannas, s., et al, Acta Ophthal, 36, 601, 1958
[5] https://www.sciencedaily.com/releases/2011/09/110912164005.htm
[6] http://www.livestrong.com/article/1001729-differencebetween-muscular-dystrophy-multiple-sclerosis/
[7] http://www.umm.edu/patiented/articles/what_gallstones_gallbladder_disease_000010_1.htm ; Watanabe, N., Arch. Surg., 85, 136, 1962
[8] http://www.sciencedaily.com/releases/2006/09/060915205102.htm
[9] http://www.ncbi.nlm.nih.gov/pubmed/18787911
[10] http://www.webmd.com/heart-disease/guide/heart-diseaselower-cholesterol-risk
[11] http://www.springerlink.com/content/ntk010354r09731k/
[12] Gross, P., et al, NY State Journal of Med 50, 2683, 1950
[13] Vannas, s., et al, Acta Ophthal, 36, 601, 1958
[14] http://realhealthtalk.com/cholesterol_exposing_the_myth.html
[15] http://www.thefreedictionary.com/calorie
[16] Jolliff, N., et al, Postgrad. Med., 29, 569, 1961; Nutritional Rev., 14, 132, 1965; Horlick, L., Canadian med. J., 83, 1186, 1960; Horlick, L., Canadian med. J., 85, 1127, 1961; Albrink, M.J., Arch. Int. Med., 109, 345,1962
[17] Hand, D.B. J. Am. Med. Assoc., 181, 411,1962; Horlick, L., Lab. Invest. 8, 723, 1959
[18] Haust, H. L., et al, Arch. BioCHem. 78, 367, 1958; Lewis, B., Lancet 1, 1090, 1958; Mead J. F., et al, J. of Biol. Chem. 229, 575, 1957
[19] Morrison, L. M., Geriatrics 13, 12, 1958
[20] Wilkins, J.A., et al, Candian J. of BioChem. Physiol., 40, 1079, 1091, 1962; Sebrell, W.H., et al, J. Am. Diet. Asson., 40, 403, 1962; Mann, G.V., Circul. Res. 9, 838, 1961; Reiser, R., et al, Circul. Res. 7, 833, 1959
[21] http://realhealthtalk.com/cholesterol_exposing_the_myth.html
[22] http://healthyeating.sfgate.com/distinguish-betweensaturated-unsaturated-fats-7667.html
[23] http://www.fda.gov/Food/GuidanceComplianceRegulatoryInformation/GuidanceDocuments/FoodLabelingNutrition/ucm053479.htm
[24] Kingsbury, K., J. of CLin. Sci. 22, 161, 1962; Antonis, A.,

Essential Fatty Acids, Academic Press, NY, NY, 1958; Lewis, B., Lancet 2, 71, 1958
[25] https://www.drdavidwilliams.com/ldl-hdl-cholesterol/
[26] http://www.sciencedirect.com/science/article/pii/0021968176900722
[27] Dahl,L.R.,et al, Fed. Proc., 1954
[28] https://www.ncbi.nlm.nih.gov/pubmed/8935479
[29] Kimura,D.,et al, J. Vitaminol. 4,310, 1958
[30] Wormersley, R.A. et al J. Clin. Invest.,34, 456, 1958
[31] Fourman, P., Clin. Sel., 13, 93, 1954
[32] Wormersley, R.A. et al J. Clin. Invest.,34, 456, 1958
[33] http://www.webmd.boots.com/heart-disease/guide/oedema
[34] https://www.webmd.com/a-to-z-guides/hyperkalemia-causes-symptoms-treatments#1
[35] http://www.healthcommunities.com/electrolyte-imbalance/too-much-potassium-too-little-potassium_jhmwp.shtml
[36] http://www.groceteria.com/about/a-quick-history-of-thesupermarket/
[37] http://en.wikipedia.org/wiki/Food_processing
[38] http://www.salon.com/2012/03/03/the_rise_and_fall_of_white_bread/
[39] http://blogs.creighton.edu/heaney/2013/11/18/pellagra-andthe-four-ds/
[40] https://www.uab.edu/reynolds/pellagra/history
[41] https://www.accessdata.fda.gov/scripts/cdrh/cfdocs/cfcfr/CFRSearch.cfm?fr=101.9
[42] Vannas, s., et al, Acta Ophthal, 36, 601, 1958
[43] http://diabetes.diabetesjournals.org/content/51/12/3353.full
[44] http://www.cdc.gov/arthritis/data_statistics/state.htm
[45] http://drfeder.com/scripts/articles_printerFriendly.php?articleID=317
[46] http://www.cancer.org/acs/groups/cid/documents/webcontent/002048-pdf.pdf
[47] http://www.naturalnews.com/024694_oil_food_oils.html
[48] http://www.healthy-eating-politics.com/vegetable-oil.html
[49] https://en.wikipedia.org/wiki/Arachidonic_acid
[50] https://en.wikipedia.org/wiki/Linoleic_acid
[51] https://en.wikipedia.org/wiki/Linolenic_acid
[52] Brown, J.B., Nutritional Rev. 17, 321, 1959
[53] Swell, L., et al, Proc. Soc. Exp. Biol. Med. 104, 325, 1960
[54] Nutritional Rev.,20,220, 1962; King, C.G., J. Amer. Diet.
[55] Gordon, H. et al, Nature 180, 923, 1957; Hellman, L, et al J. Clin. Invest. 36, 898, 1957; Deykin, D., et al, J. Biol. Chem. 237, 3649, 1962
[56] Deykin, D., et al, J. Biol. Chem. 237, 3649, 1962;Peifer, J. G., et al, J. Nutrition, 68, 155, 1959; Merrill, J.M., Circul. Res. 7, 709, 1959
[57] https://www.reference.com/science/difference-betweenlinoleic-linolenic-acid-1661b7ceb0c1f093

[58] Capeci, N.E., et al, Am. J. Med. 26, 76, 1959
[59] King, C.G., J. Amer. Diet. Assoc. 42, 199, 1963; Haust, H.L., et al, J. Nutrition, 81, 13, 1963; Ahrens E.H., Jr., et al, Lencat 1, 115, 1959; Capeci, N.E., et al, Am. J. Med. 26, 76, 1959
[60] http://www.wisegeek.com/what-are-fatty-acids.htm#
[61] http://www.fda.gov/Food/GuidanceComplianceRegulatoryInformation/GuidanceDocuments/FoodLabelingNutrition/ucm053479.htm
[62] https://www.youtube.com/watch?v=i3UiG0VpVI4&t=20s
[63] Nutritional Rev., 20, 220, 1962
[64] Horlick, L., Circulation 10, 30, 1956; Duff, G.L., et al, Am. J. Med., 11, 92, 1951; Adlersburg, D., et al, J. Nutritional Rev., 25, 255, 1943
[65] Nutritional Rev., 20, 220, 1962; Byers, S.O., Am. J. Clin. Nutrition, 6, 638, 1958;
[66] Artom, C., Am. J. Clin. Nutrition, 6, 221, 1958
[67] Adlersburg, D., et al, Clin. Chem., 1, 18, 1955; Thannhauser, S.J., et al, J. Bio. Chem., 129, 717, 1939
[68] Adlersburg, D., et al, Clin. Chem., 1, 18, 1955; Horlick, L., Circulation 10, 30, 1956
[69] Davies, D.F., Clin. Sci., 17, 563, 1958; Ahrems, E.H. et al, J. Exp. Med., 90, 409, 1949; Leathes, J.B., Lancet 1, 1019, 1925
[70] Hirsch, E.F., et al, Physiological Rev., 23, 185, 1943
[71] Hirsch, E.F., et al, Physiological Rev., 23, 185, 1943
[72] Kesten, H.D., et al, Proc. Soc. Exp. Biol. Med., 49, 71, 1941
[73] Kesten, H.D., et al, Proc. Soc. Exp. Biol. Med., 49, 71, 1941
[74] Ladd, A.T., et al, Fed. Proc. 8, 360, 1949
[75] Artom, C., Am. J. Clin. Nutrition, 6, 221, 1958; Havel, R.J., J. Clin. Invest., 36, 848, 1957; Freidman, M., et al, Am. J. Physiol. 186, 13, 1956; Walker, W.J., Am. J. Med. 14, 654, 1953
[76] Havel, R.J., J. Clin. Invest., 36, 848, 1957; Walker, W.J., Am. J. Med. 14, 654, 1953
[77] http://www.brainfacts.org/brain-anatomy-and-function/anatomy/2015/myelin
[78] Friedman, M., et al, Proc. Soc. Exp. Biol. Med., 95, 586, 1957
[79] Friedman, M., et al, Gerontology, 10, 60, 1955; Byers, S.O., Am. J. Clin. Nutrition, 6, 638, 1958; Friedman, M., et al, Am. J. Physiol. 186, 13, 1956
[80] https://assets.adm.com/Products-And-Services/Food-Ingredients/Lecithin/Lecithin-Candy-and-Confectionery.pdf
[81] http://www.soyinfocenter.com/HSS/lecithin2.php
[82] Zierler, m. et al, Ann. NY, Academy of Sci., 52, 180, 1949

[83] Houchim, O.B., et al, J. of Bio. Chem.,146, 309, 313, 1942
[84] DeNicola, P., Inter. Congress Vit E, 1955
[85] http://www.sosdietbook.com/index.php?page=Low_Fat_Diet_Myths ; Horlick, L., Canadian med. J., 83, 1186, 1960
[86] Eastwood, G., et al, J. Am. Diet. Assoc. 42, 518, 1963
[87] Siperstein, M.D., et al, J. Biol. Chem. 210, 181, 1954; Bremer, J., Biochem. J. 63, 507,1956
[88] Jones, E.A., et al, J. Lab. Clin. Med., 52, 667, 1958; Karvinen, E. et al, J. Applied Physiol., 11, 143, 1957; Gordon, H., Lancet, 2, 244, 1958; Conner, W.E. et al, J. Lab. Clin. Med., 57, 3331, 1961
[89] Dock, W., Am. J. Clin. Nutr. 5, 674, 1957; Dock, W., Am. J. Clin. Nutr. 6, 171, 1958
[90] Mead, J.F. et al, J. Biol. Chem., 229, 575, 1957; Sharper, A.G., Am. Heart J., 63, 437, 1962;
[91] http://dictionary.reference.com/browse/metabolic?s=t

www.ingramcontent.com/pod-product-compliance
Lightning Source LLC
Chambersburg PA
CBHW030532220526
45463CB00007B/2800